The Ultimate Air Fryer Cooking Guide

Easy And Delicious Air Fryer Recipes For Everyone

Ellie Sloan

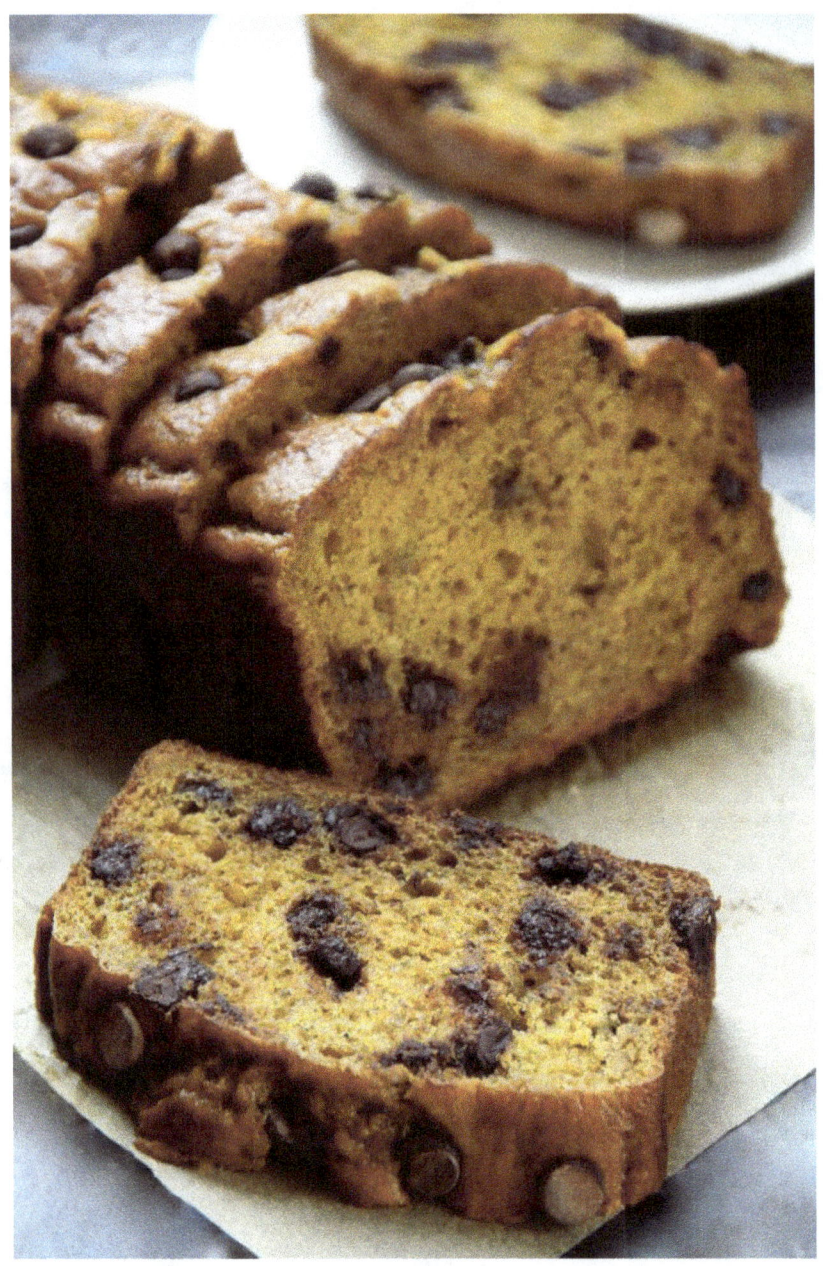

© Copyright 2020 - All rights reserved.

The content contained within this book may not be reproduced, duplicated or transmitted without direct written permission from the author or the publisher.

Under no circumstances will any blame or legal responsibility be held against the publisher, or author, for any damages, reparation, or monetary loss due to the information contained within this book. Either directly or indirectly.

Legal Notice:

This book is copyright protected. This book is only for personal use. You cannot amend, distribute, sell, use, quote or paraphrase any part, or the content within this book, without the consent of the author or publisher.

Disclaimer Notice:

Please note the information contained within this document is for educational and entertainment purposes only. All effort has been executed to present accurate, up to date, and reliable, complete information. No warranties of any kind are declared or implied. Readers acknowledge that the author is not engaging in the rendering of legal, financial, medical or professional advice. The content within this book has been derived from various sources. Please consult a licensed professional before attempting any techniques outlined in this book.

By reading this document, the reader agrees that under no circumstances is the author responsible for any losses, direct or indirect, which are incurred as a result of the use of information contained within this document, including, but not limited to, — errors, omissions, or inaccuracies.

Table of contents

Stuffed Jalapeno 7

Garlicky Bok Choy 9

Chia Seed Crackers 10

Baked Eggplant Chips 12

Flax Seed Chips 14

Salted Hazelnuts 16

Baguette Bread 18

Yogurt Bread 20

Sunflower Seed Bread 23

Date Bread 25

Date & Walnut Bread 27

Brown Sugar Banana Bread 30

Cinnamon Banana Bread 32

Banana & Walnut Bread 34

Banana & Raisin Bread 37

3-Ingredients Banana Bread 39

Yogurt Banana Bread 41

Sour Cream Banana Bread 43

Peanut Butter Banana Bread 45

Chocolate Banana Bread 48

Allspice Chicken Wings 50

Friday Night Pineapple Sticky Ribs 52

Egg Roll Wrapped with Cabbage and Prawns 54

Sesame Garlic Chicken Wings 56

Savory Chicken Nuggets with Parmesan Cheese 59

Butternut Squash with Thyme 61

Chicken Breasts in Golden Crumb 63

Yogurt Chicken Tacos 65

Flawless Kale Chips 67

Vermicelli Noodles & Vegetables Rolls 69

Cheese Fish Balls 71

Beef Balls with Mixed Herbs 73

Roasted Pumpkin Seeds 75

Buttery Parmesan Broccoli Florets 77

Spicy Chickpeas 79

Roasted Peanuts 81

Roasted Cashews 83

French Fries 84

Zucchini Fries 86

Spicy Carrot Fries 88

Cinnamon Carrot Fries 90

Squash Fries 91

Avocado Fries 93

Dill Pickle Fries 95

Mozzarella Sticks 97

Tortilla Chips 99

Sky-High Roasted Corn 101

Ravishing Air-Fried Carrots with Honey Glaze 102

Flaming Buffalo Cauliflower Bites 104

Pleasant Air-Fried Eggplant.. 106

Stuffed Jalapeno

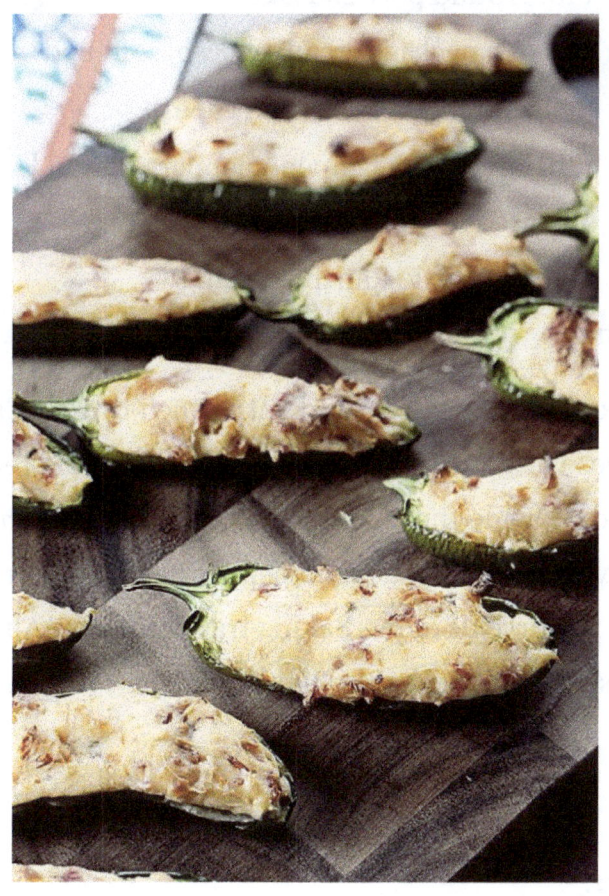

Preparation Time: 10 minutes

Cooking Time: 10 minutes

Servings: 4

Ingredients:

- 1 lb. ground pork sausage
- 1 (8 oz.) package cream cheese, softened
- 1 cup shredded Parmesan cheese
- 1 lb. large fresh jalapeno peppers halved lengthwise and seeded
- 1 (8 oz.) bottle Ranch dressing

Directions:

Mix pork sausage ground with ranch dressing and cream cheese in a bowl. Cut the jalapeno in half and remove their seeds. Divide the cream cheese mixture into the jalapeno halves. Place the jalapeno pepper in a baking tray that fits the Air Fryer. Set the Baking tray inside the Air Fryer and close the lid. Select the Bake mode at 350°F temperature for 10 minutes. Serve warm.

Nutrition:

Calories 168, Protein 9.4g, Carbs 12.1g, Fat 21.2g

Garlicky Bok Choy

Preparation Time: 10 minutes

Cooking Time: 6 minutes

Servings: 2

Ingredients:

- Bunches baby bok choy
- spray oil
- 1 tsp. garlic powder

Directions:

Toss bok choy with garlic powder and spread them in the Air Fryer basket. Spray them with cooking oil. Set the Air Fryer basket inside the Air Fryer and close the lid. Select the Air Fry mode at 350°F temperature for 6 minutes. Serve fresh.

Nutrition:

Calories 81, Protein 0.4g, Carbs 4.7g, Fat 8.3g

Chia Seed Crackers

Preparation Time: 15 minutes

Cooking Time: 45 minutes

Servings: 48

Ingredients:

- 1 Cup raw chia seed
- 3/4 Tsp. salt
- 1/4 Tsp. garlic powder
- 1/4 Tsp. onion powder
- 1 Cup cold water

Directions:

1. Put the chia seeds in a bowl. Add salt, garlic powder, and onion powder.
2. Pour into the water. Stir. Cover with plastic wrap. Store in the fridge overnight. Preheat the Air Fryer to 200°F. Cover the baking sheet with a silicone mat or parchment. Transfer the soaked linseed to a prepared baking sheet. Scatter it out with a spatula in a thin, flat rectangle about 1 cm thick. Rate the rectangle in about 32 small rectangles.

Bake in the preheated Air Fryer toaster oven up to the chia seeds have darkened and contract slightly, about 3 hours. Let it cool. Break individual cookies.

Nutrition:

Calories 120, Fat 3.9g, Carbs 1.9g, Protein 1.9g

Baked Eggplant Chips

Preparation Time: 5 minutes

Cooking Time: 8 minutes

Servings: 4

Ingredients:

- Medium eggplant, cut into 1/4-inch slices
- 1/2 Cup crushed cornflakes.
- 1/8 Tsp. ground black pepper
- Tbsp. grated goat cheese
- Egg whites

Directions:

1. Preheat the Air Fryer to 400°F. Mix the crushed cornflakes, pepper and goat cheese in a small container. Set aside the egg whites in a different container. Dip the eggplant slices in the egg white and cover the crushed cornflakes mixture. Place on a greased baking pan that fits the Air Dryer.
2. Air fry for 3 minutes, then turn and cook bake for another 3 to 5 minutes until golden yellow and crispy.

Nutrition:

Calories 92, Fat 2.1g, Carbs 13.9g, Protein 5.9g

Flax Seed Chips

Preparation Time: 5 minutes

Cooking Time: 8 minutes

Servings: 4

Ingredients:

- 1 Cup almond flour
- 1/2 Cup flax seeds
- 1 1/2 Tsp.s seasoned salt
- 1 Tsp. sea salt
- 1/2 Cup water

Directions:

1. Preheat the Air Fryer to 300°F. Combine almond flour, flax seeds, 1 1/2 tsp.s seasoned salt and sea salt in a container; Stir in the water up to the dough is completely mixed. Shape the dough into narrow size slices the size of a bite and place them on a pan that fits the Air Dryer. Sprinkle the rounds with seasoned salt. Bake in preheated Air Fryer up to crispy, about 8 minutes. Cool fully and store in an airtight box or in a sealed bag.

Nutrition:

Calories 126.9, Fat 6.1g, Carbs 15.9g, Protein 2.9g

Salted Hazelnuts

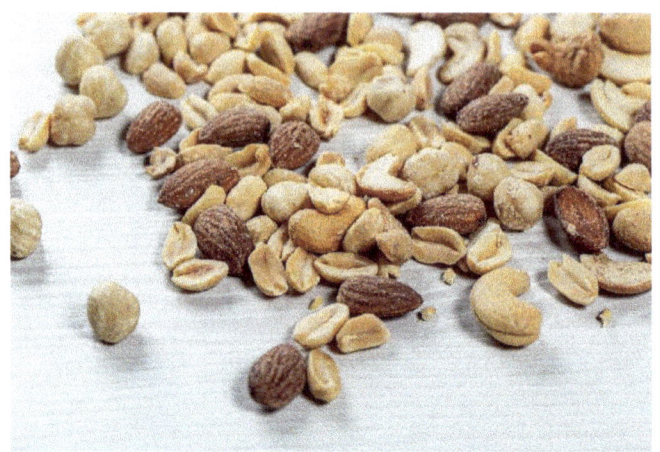

Preparation Time: 15 minutes

Cooking Time: 6 minutes

Servings: 8

Ingredients:

- Cups dry roasted Hazelnuts, no salt added
- Tbsp. coconut oil
- 1 Tsp. garlic powder
- 1 Sprig fresh Thyme, chopped
- 1 1/2 Tsp.s salt

Directions:

Preheat the Air Fryer to 320°F. Mix the Hazelnuts, coconut oil, garlic powder and thyme in a bowl until the nuts are fully covered. Sprinkle with salt. Spread evenly on a baking sheet. Bake in the preheated Air Fryer for 6 minutes.

Nutrition:

Calories 237, Fat 21.3g, Carbs 5.9g, Protein 7.4g

Baguette Bread

Preparation Time: 15 minutes

Cooking Time: 8 minutes

Servings: 8

Ingredients:

- ¾ cup warm water
- ¾ tsp. quick yeast
- ½ tsp. demerara sugar
- 1 cup bread flour
- ½ cup whole-wheat flour
- ½ cup oat flour
- 1¼ tsp.s salt

Directions:

1. In a large bowl, place the water and sprinkle with yeast and sugar. Set aside for 5 minutes or until foamy.
2. Add the bread flour and salt mix until a stiff dough form.

3. Put the dough onto a floured surface and with your hands, knead until smooth and elastic. Shape the dough into a ball.
4. Place the dough into a slightly oiled bowl and turn to coat well.
5. With a plastic wrap, cover the bowl and place in a warm place for about 1 hour or until doubled in size.
6. With your hands, punch down the dough and form into a long slender loaf.
7. Place the loaf onto a lightly greased baking sheet and set aside in warm place, uncovered, for about 30 minutes
8. Heat the Air Fryer 450°F.
9. Carefully, arrange the dough onto the "Wire Rack" and insert in the Air Fryer.
10. Air Fry for 8 minutes.
11. Carefully, invert the bread onto wire rack to cool completely before slicing.
12. Cut the bread into desired-sized slices and serve.

Nutrition:

Calories 114, Fat 0.8g, Carbs 22.8g, Protein 3.8g

Yogurt Bread

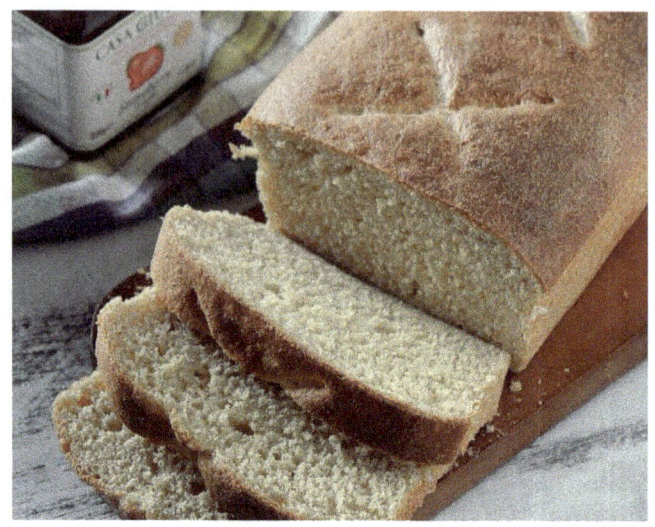

Preparation Time: 20 minutes

Cooking Time: 20 minutes

Servings: 10

Ingredients:

- 1½ cups warm water, divided
- 1½ tsp.s active dry yeast
- 1 tsp. sugar
- 3 cups all-purpose flour
- 1 cup plain Greek yogurt

- 2 tsp.s kosher salt

Directions:

1. Add ½ cup of the warm water, yeast and sugar in the bowl of a stand mixer, fitted with the dough hook attachment and mix well.
2. Set aside for about 5 minutes
3. Add the flour, yogurt, and salt and mix on medium-low speed until the dough comes together.
4. Then, mix on medium speed for 5 minutes
5. Place the dough into a bowl.
6. With a plastic wrap, cover the bowl and place in a warm place for about 2-3 hours or until doubled in size.
7. Transfer the dough onto a lightly floured surface and shape into a smooth ball.
8. Place the dough onto a greased parchment paper-lined rack.
9. With a kitchen towel, cover the dough and let rest for 15 minutes
10. With a very sharp knife, cut a 4x½-inch deep cut down the center of the dough.
11. Preheat the Air Fryer at 325°F.

12. Carefully, arrange the dough onto the "Wire Rack" and insert in the Air Fryer. Cook for 20 minutes.
13. Carefully, invert the bread onto wire rack to cool completely before slicing.
14. Cut the bread into desired-sized slices and serve.

Nutrition:

Calories 157, Fat 0.7g, Carbs 31g, Protein 5.5g

Sunflower Seed Bread

Preparation Time: 15 minutes

Cooking Time: 18 minutes

Servings: 6

Ingredients:

- 2/3 cup whole-wheat flour
- 2/3 cup plain flour
- 1/3 cup sunflower seeds
- ½ sachet instant yeast
- 1 tsp. salt
- 2/3-1 cup lukewarm water

Directions:

1. In a bowl, mix together the flours, sunflower seeds, yeast, and salt.
2. Slowly, add in the water, stirring continuously until a soft dough ball form.
3. Now, move the dough onto a lightly floured surface and knead for about 5 minutes using your hands.
4. Make a ball from the dough and place into a bowl.

5. With a plastic wrap, cover the bowl and place at a warm place for about 30 minutes
6. Grease a cake pan that fits the Air Fryer.
7. Coat the top of dough with water and place into the prepared cake pan.
8. Preheat the Air Fryer at 390°F.
9. Arrange the pan in the Air Fryer basket and insert in the oven. Cook for 18 minutes.
10. Place the pan onto a wire rack to cool for about 10 minutes
11. Carefully, invert the bread onto wire rack to cool completely before slicing.
12. Cut the bread into desired-sized slices and serve.

Nutrition:

Calories 132, Fat 1.7g, Carbs 24.4g, Protein 4.9g

Date Bread

Preparation Time: 15 minutes

Cooking Time: 22 minutes

Servings: 10

Ingredients:

- 2½ cup dates, pitted and chopped
- ¼ cup butter
- 1 cup hot water
- 1½ cups flour
- ½ cup brown sugar
- 1 tsp. baking powder
- 1 tsp. baking soda
- ½ tsp. salt
- 1 egg

Directions:

1. In a large bowl, add the dates, butter and top with the hot water.
2. Set aside for about 5 minutes

3. In another bowl, mix together the flour, brown sugar, baking powder, baking soda, and salt.
4. In the same bowl of dates, mix well the flour mixture, and egg.
5. Grease a baking pan.
6. Place the mixture into the prepared pan.
7. Preheat the Air Fryer at 340°F.
8. Arrange the pan in Air Fryer basket and insert in the oven. Cook for about 22 minutes.
9. Place the pan onto a wire rack to cool for about 10 minutes
10. Carefully, invert the bread onto wire rack to cool completely before slicing.
11. Cut the bread into desired-sized slices and serve.

Nutrition:

Calories 269, Fat 5.4g, Carbs 55.1g, Protein 3.6g

Date & Walnut Bread

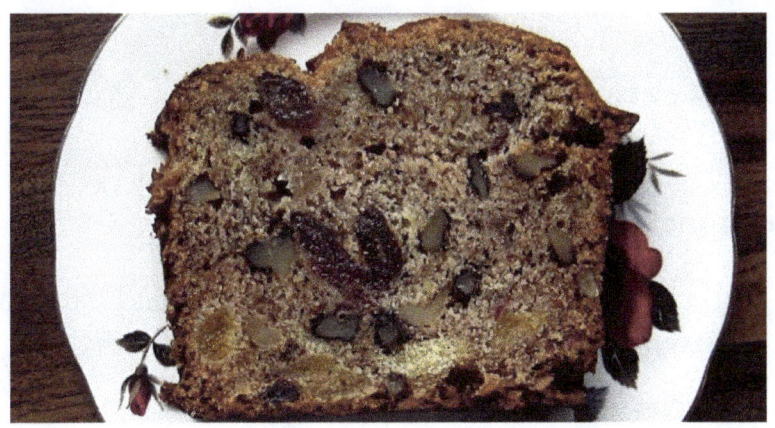

Preparation Time: 15 minutes

Cooking Time: 35 minutes

Servings: 5

Ingredients:

- 1 cup dates, pitted and sliced
- ¾ cup walnuts, chopped
- 1 tbsp. instant coffee powder
- 1 tbsp. hot water
- 1¼ cups plain flour
- ¼ tsp. salt
- ½ tsp. baking powder

- ½ tsp. baking soda
- ½ cup condensed milk
- ½ cup butter, softened
- ½ tsp. vanilla essence

Directions:

1. In a large bowl, add the dates, butter and top with the hot water.
2. Set aside for about 30 minutes
3. Dry out well and set aside.
4. In a small bowl, add the coffee powder and hot water and mix well.
5. In a large bowl, mix together the flour, baking powder, baking soda and salt.
6. In another large bowl, add the condensed milk and butter and beat until smooth.
7. Add the flour mixture, coffee mixture and vanilla essence and mix until well combined.
8. Fold in dates and ½ cup of walnut.
9. Line a baking pan with a lightly greased parchment paper.
10. Place the mixture into the prepared pan and sprinkle with the remaining walnuts.
11. Preheat the Air Fryer at 320°F.

12. Arrange the pan in Air Fryer basket and insert in the oven. Cook for 35 minutes.
13. Place the pan onto a wire rack to cool for about 10 minutes
14. Carefully, invert the bread onto wire rack to cool completely before slicing.
15. Cut the bread into desired-sized slices and serve.

Nutrition:

Calories 593, Fat 32.6g, Carbs 69.4g, Protein 11.2g

Brown Sugar Banana Bread

Preparation Time: 15 minutes

Cooking Time: 30 minutes

Servings: 4

Ingredients:

- 1 egg
- 1 ripe banana, peeled and mashed
- ¼ cup milk
- 2 tbsp. canola oil
- 2 tbsp. brown sugar
- ¾ cup plain flour
- ½ tsp. baking soda

Directions:

1. Line a very small baking pan with a greased parchment paper.
2. In a small bowl, add the egg and banana and beat well.
3. Add the milk, oil and sugar and beat until well combined.

4. Add the flour and baking soda and mix until just combined.
5. Place the mixture into prepared pan.
6. Preheat the Air Fryer at 320°F.
7. Arrange the pan in Air Fryer basket and insert in the oven. Cook for 30 minutes.
8. Place the pan onto a wire rack to cool for about 10 minutes
9. Carefully, invert the bread onto wire rack to cool completely before slicing.
10. Cut the bread into desired-sized slices and serve.

Nutrition:

Calories 214, Fat 8.7g, Carbs 29.9g, Protein 4.6g

Cinnamon Banana Bread

Preparation Time: 15 minutes

Cooking Time: 20 minutes

Servings: 8

Ingredients:

- 1 1/3 cups flour
- 2/3 cup sugar
- 1 tsp. baking soda
- 1 tsp. baking powder
- 1 tsp. ground cinnamon
- 1 tsp. salt
- ½ cup milk
- ½ cup olive oil
- 3 bananas, peeled and sliced

Directions:

1. In the bowl of a stand mixer, add all the ingredients and mix well.
2. Grease a loaf pan.
3. Place the mixture into the prepared pan.

4. Preheat the Air Fryer at 320°F.
5. Arrange the pan in Air Fryer basket and insert in the oven. Cook for 20 minutes.
6. Place the pan onto a wire rack to cool for about 10 minutes
7. Carefully, invert the bread onto wire rack to cool completely before slicing.
8. Cut the bread into desired-sized slices and serve.

Nutrition:

Calories 295, Fat 13.3g, Carbs 44g, Protein 3.1g

Banana & Walnut Bread

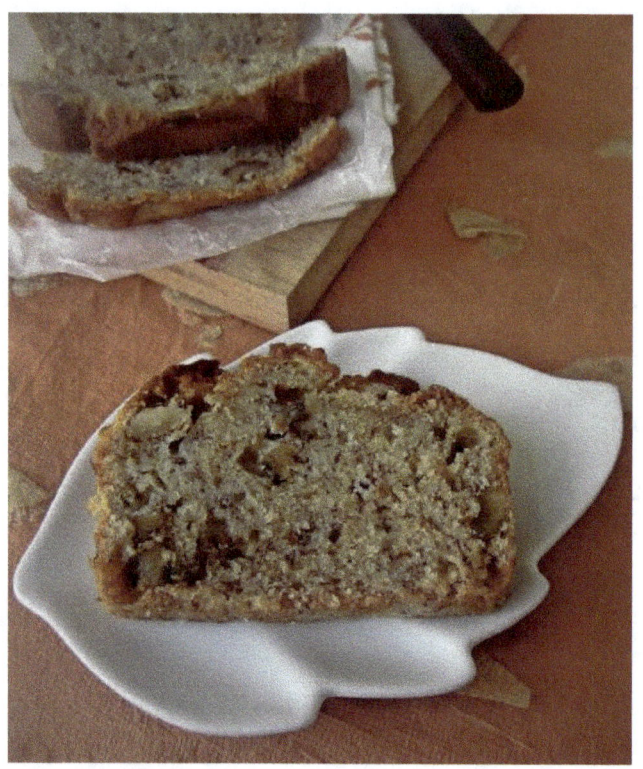

Preparation Time: 15 minutes

Cooking Time: 25 minutes

Servings: 10

Ingredients:

- 1½ cups self-rising flour

- ¼ tsp. bicarbonate of soda
- 5 tbsp. plus 1 tsp. butter
- 2/3 cup plus ½ tbsp. caster sugar
- 2 medium eggs
- 3½ oz. walnuts, chopped
- 2 cups bananas, peeled and mashed

Directions:

1. In a bowl, mix together the flour and bicarbonate of soda.
2. In another bowl, add the butter, and sugar and beat until pale and fluffy.
3. Add the eggs, one at a time along with a little flour and mix well.
4. Stir in the remaining flour and walnuts. Add the bananas and mix until well combined.
5. Grease a loaf pan. Place the mixture into the prepared pan.
6. Preheat the Air Fryer at 350°F.
7. Arrange the pan in Air Fryer basket and insert in the oven. Cook for 10 minutes.
8. After 10 minutes of cooking, set the temperature at 320°F for 15 minutes

9. Place the pan onto a wire rack to cool for about 10 minutes
10. Carefully, invert the bread onto wire rack to cool completely before slicing.
11. Cut the bread into desired-sized slices and serve.

Nutrition:

Calories 270, Fat 12.8g, Carbs 35.5g, Protein 5.8g

Banana & Raisin Bread

Preparation Time: 15 minutes

Cooking Time: 40 minutes

Servings: 6

Ingredients:

- 1½ cups cake flour
- 1 tsp. baking soda
- ½ tsp. ground cinnamon
- Salt, to taste
- ½ cup vegetable oil
- 2 eggs
- ½ cup sugar
- ½ tsp. vanilla extract
- 3 medium bananas, peeled and mashed
- ½ cup raisins, chopped finely

Directions:

1. In a large bowl, mix together the flour, baking soda, cinnamon, and salt.
2. In another bowl, beat well eggs and oil.

3. Add the sugar, vanilla extract, and bananas and beat until well combined.
4. Add the flour mixture and stir until just combined.
5. Place the mixture into a lightly greased baking pan and sprinkle with raisins.
6. With a piece of foil, cover the pan loosely.
7. Preheat the Air Fryer at 300°F.
8. Arrange the pan in Air Fryer basket and insert in the oven. Cook for 30 minutes.
9. After 30 minutes of cooking, set the temperature to 285°F for 10 minutes
10. Place the pan onto a wire rack to cool for about 10 minutes
11. Carefully, invert the bread onto wire rack to cool completely before slicing.
12. Cut the bread into desired-sized slices and serve.

Nutrition:

Calories 448, Fat 20.2, Carbs 63.9g, Protein 6.1g

3-Ingredients Banana Bread

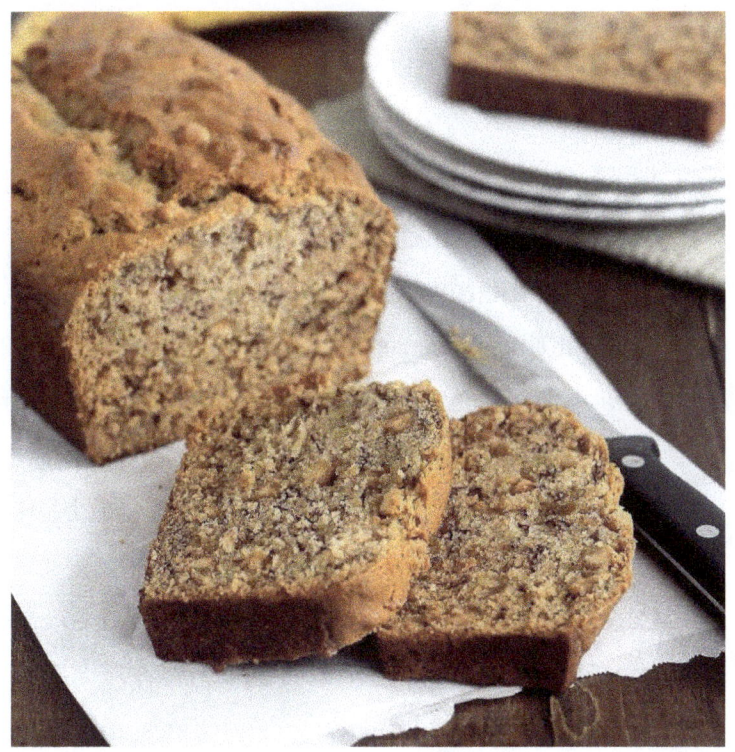

Preparation Time: 10 minutes

Cooking Time: 20 minutes:

Servings: 6

Ingredients:

- 2 (6.4-oz.) banana muffin mix

- 1 cup water
- 1 ripe banana, peeled and mashed

Directions:

1. In a bowl, add all the ingredients and with a whisk, mix until well combined.
2. Place the mixture into a lightly greased loaf pan.
3. Preheat the Air Fryer at 360°F.
4. Arrange the pan in Air Fryer basket and insert in the oven. Cook for 20 minutes:.
5. Place the pan onto a wire rack to cool for about 10 minutes
6. Carefully, invert the bread onto wire rack to cool completely before slicing.
7. Cut the bread into desired-sized slices and serve.

Nutrition:

Calories 144, Fat 3.8g, Carbs 25.5g, Protein 1.9g

Yogurt Banana Bread

Preparation Time: 15 minutes

Cooking Time: 28 minutes

Servings: 5

Ingredients:

- 1 medium very ripe banana, peeled and mashed
- 1 large egg
- 1 tbsp. canola oil
- 1 tbsp. plain Greek yogurt
- ¼ tsp. pure vanilla extract
- ½ cup all-purpose flour
- ¼ cup granulated white sugar
- ¼ tsp. ground cinnamon
- ¼ tsp. baking soda
- 1/8 tsp. sea salt

Directions:

1. In a bowl, add the mashed banana, egg, oil, yogurt and vanilla and beat until well combined.

2. Add the flour, sugar, baking soda, cinnamon and salt and mix until just combined.
3. Place the mixture into a lightly greased mini loaf pan.
4. Preheat the Air Fryer at 350°F.
5. Arrange the pan in Air Fryer basket and insert in the oven. Cook for 28 minutes.
6. Place the pan onto a wire rack to cool for about 10 minutes
7. Carefully, invert the bread onto wire rack to cool completely before slicing.
8. Cut the bread into desired-sized slices and serve.

Nutrition:

Calories 145, Fat 4g, Carbs 25g, Protein 3g

Sour Cream Banana Bread

Preparation Time: 15 minutes

Cooking Time: 37 minutes

Servings: 8

Ingredients:

- ¾ cup all-purpose flour
- ¼ tsp. baking soda
- ¼ tsp. salt
- 2 ripe bananas, peeled and mashed
- ½ cup granulated sugar
- ¼ cup sour cream
- ¼ cup vegetable oil
- 1 large egg
- ½ tsp. pure vanilla extract

Directions:

1. In a large bowl, mix together the flour, baking soda and salt.
2. In another bowl, add the bananas, egg, sugar, sour cream, oil and vanilla and beat until well combined.

3. Add the flour mixture and mix until just combined.
4. Preheat the Air Fryer at 310°F.
5. Arrange the pan in Air Fryer basket and insert in the oven. Cook for 37 minutes.
6. Place the pan onto a wire rack to cool for about 10 minutes
7. Carefully, invert the bread onto wire rack to cool completely before slicing.
8. Cut the bread into desired-sized slices and serve.

Nutrition:

Calories 201, Fat 9.2g, Carbs 28.6g, Protein 2.6g

Peanut Butter Banana Bread

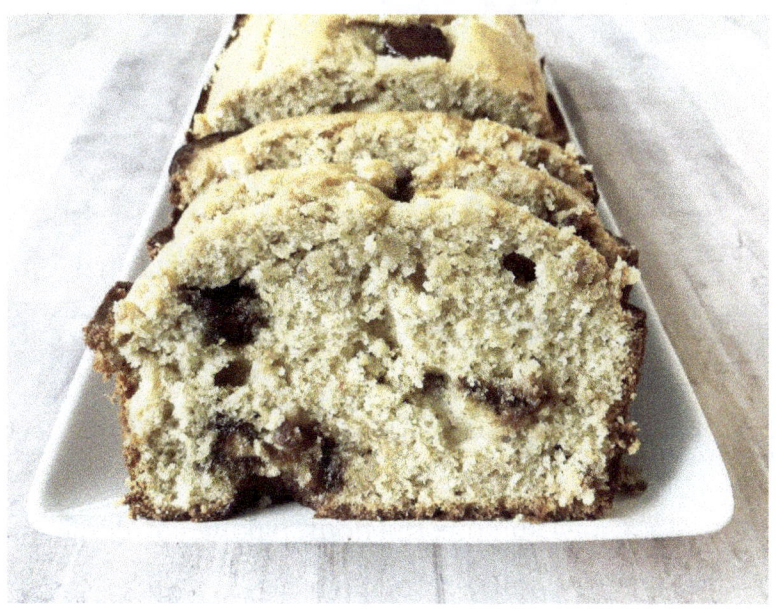

Preparation Time: 15 minutes

Cooking Time: 40 minutes

Servings: 6

Ingredients:

- 1 cup plus 1 tbsp. all-purpose flour
- ¼ tsp. baking soda
- 1 tsp. baking powder
- ¼ tsp. salt

- 1 large egg
- 1/3 cup granulated sugar
- ¼ cup canola oil
- 2 tbsp. creamy peanut butter
- 2 tbsp. sour cream
- 1 tsp. vanilla extract
- 2 medium ripe bananas, peeled and mashed
- ¾ cup walnuts, roughly chopped

Directions:

1. In a bowl and mix the flour, baking powder, baking soda, and salt together.
2. In another large bowl, add the egg, sugar, oil, peanut butter, sour cream, and vanilla extract and beat until well combined.
3. Add the bananas and beat until well combined. Add the flour mixture and mix until just combined.
4. Gently, fold in the walnuts. Place the mixture into a lightly greased pan.
5. Preheat the Air Fryer at 330°F.
6. Arrange the pan in Air Fryer basket and insert in the oven. Cook for 40 minutes.
7. Place the pan onto a wire rack to cool for about 10 minutes

8. Carefully, invert the bread onto wire rack to cool completely before slicing.
9. Cut the bread into desired-sized slices and serve.

Nutrition:

Calories 384, Fat 23g, Carbs 39.3g, Protein 8.9g

Chocolate Banana Bread

Preparation Time: 15 minutes

Cooking Time: 20 minutes:

Servings: 8

Ingredients:

- 2 cups flour
- ½ tsp. baking soda
- ½ tsp. baking powder
- ½ tsp. salt
- ¾ cup sugar
- 1/3 cup butter, softened
- 3 eggs
- 1 tbsp. vanilla extract
- 1 cup milk
- ½ cup bananas, peeled and mashed
- 1 cup chocolate chips

Directions:

1. In a bowl, mix together the flour, baking soda, baking powder, and salt.

2. In another large bowl, add the butter, and sugar and beat until light and fluffy.
3. Add the eggs, and vanilla extract and whisk until well combined.
4. Add the flour mixture and mix until well combined.
5. Add the milk, and mashed bananas and mix well.
6. Gently, fold in the chocolate chips. Place the mixture into a lightly greased loaf pan.
7. Preheat the Air Fryer at 360°F.
8. Arrange the pan in Air Fryer basket and insert in the oven. Cook for 20 minutes.
9. Place the pan onto a wire rack to cool for about 10 minutes Carefully, invert the bread onto wire rack to cool completely before slicing.
10. Cut the bread into desired-sized slices and serve.

Nutrition:

Calories, Fat 16.5g, Carbs 59.2g, Protein 8.1g

Allspice Chicken Wings

Cooking Time: 45 minutes

Serving: 8

Ingredients:

- ½ tsp. celery salt
- ½ tsp. bay leaf powder
- ½ tsp. ground black pepper
- ½ tsp. paprika
- ¼ tsp. dry mustard
- ¼ tsp. cayenne pepper
- ¼ tsp. allspice
- 2 lb. chicken wings

Directions:

1. Grease the Air Fryer basket and preheat to 340°F. In a bowl, mix celery salt, bay leaf powder, black pepper, paprika, dry mustard, cayenne pepper, and allspice. Coat the wings thoroughly in this mixture.
2. Arrange the wings in an even layer in the basket of the Air Fryer. Cook the chicken until it's no longer

pinks around the bone, for 30 minutes then, increase the temperature to 380°F and cook for 6 minutes more, until crispy on the outside.

Nutrition:

Calories 332, Fat 10.1g, Carbs 31.3g, Protein 12g

Friday Night Pineapple Sticky Ribs

Preparation Time: 10 minutes

Cooking Time: 20 minutes:

Servings: 4

Ingredients:

- 2 lb. cut spareribs
- 7 oz salad dressing
- 1 (5-oz) can pineapple juice
- 2 cups water
- Garlic salt to taste
- Salt and black pepper

Directions:

1. Sprinkle the ribs with salt and pepper, and place them in a saucepan. Pour water and cook the ribs for 12 minutes on high heat.
2. Dry out the ribs and arrange them in the fryer; sprinkle with garlic salt. Cook it for 15 minutes at 390°F.

3. Prepare the sauce by combining the salad dressing and the pineapple juice. Serve the ribs drizzled with the sauce.

Nutrition:

Calories 316, Fat 3.1g, Carbs 1.9g, Protein 5g

Egg Roll Wrapped with Cabbage and Prawns

Preparation Time: 10 minutes

Cooking Time: 40 minutes

Servings: 4

Ingredients:

- 2 tbsp. vegetable oil
- 1-inch piece fresh ginger, grated
- 1 tbsp. minced garlic
- 1 carrot, cut into strips
- ¼ cup chicken broth
- 2 tbsp. reduced-sodium soy sauce
- 1 tbsp. sugar
- 1 cup shredded Napa cabbage
- 1 tbsp. sesame oil
- 8 cooked prawns, minced
- 1 egg
- 8 egg roll wrappers

Directions:

1. In a skillet over high heat, heat vegetable oil, and cook ginger and garlic for 40 seconds, until fragrant. Stir in carrot and cook for another 2 minutes. Pour in chicken broth, soy sauce, and sugar and bring to a boil.
2. Add cabbage and let simmer until softened, for 4 minutes. Remove skillet from the heat and stir in sesame oil. Let cool for 15 minutes. Strain cabbage mixture, and fold in minced prawns. Whisk an egg in a small bowl. Fill each egg roll wrapper with prawn mixture, arranging the mixture just below the center of the wrapper.
3. Fold the bottom part over the filling and tuck under. Fold in both sides and tightly roll up. Use the whisked egg to seal the wrapper. Repeat until all egg rolls are ready. Place the rolls into a greased Air Fryer basket, spray them with oil and cook for 12 minutes at 370°F, turning once halfway through.

Nutrition:

Calories 215, Fat 7.9g, Carbs 6.7g, Protein 8g

Sesame Garlic Chicken Wings

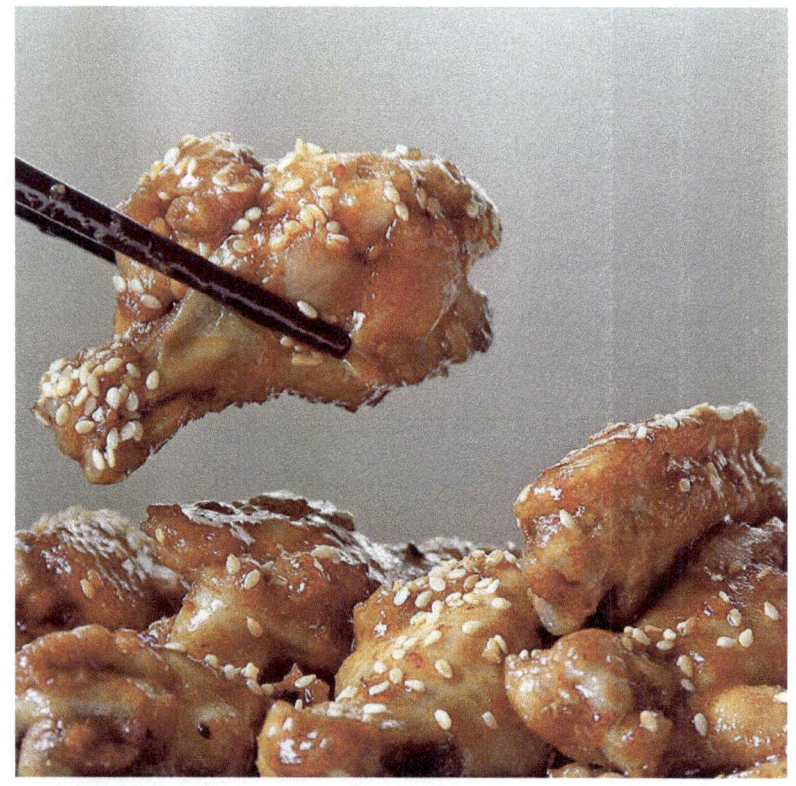

Preparation Time: 10 minutes

Cooking Time: 40 minutes

Servings: 4

Ingredients:

- 1-lb. chicken wings

- 1 cup soy sauce, divided
- ½ cup brown sugar
- ½ cup apple cider vinegar
- 2 tbsp. fresh ginger, minced
- 2 tbsp. fresh garlic, minced
- 1 tsp. finely ground black pepper
- 2 tbsp. cornstarch
- 2 tbsp. cold water
- 1 tsp. sesame seeds

Directions:

1. In a bowl, add chicken wings, and pour in half cup soy sauce. Refrigerate for 20 minutes; Dry out and pat dry. Arrange the wings in the Air Fryer and cook for 30 minutes at 380°F, turning once halfway through. Make sure you check them towards the end to avoid overcooking.
2. In a skillet and over medium heat, stir sugar, half cup soy sauce, vinegar, ginger, garlic, and black pepper. Cook until sauce has reduced slightly, about 4 to 6 minutes
3. Dissolve 2 tbsp. of cornstarch in cold water, in a bowl, and stir in the slurry into the sauce, until it thickens,

for 2 minutes. Pour the sauce over wings and sprinkle with sesame seeds.

Nutrition:

Calories 413, Fat 8.3g, Carbs 7g, Protein 8.3g

Savory Chicken Nuggets with Parmesan Cheese

Preparation Time: 5 minutes

Cooking Time: 20 minutes:

Servings: 4

Ingredients:

- 1 lb. chicken breast, boneless, skinless, cubed
- ½ tsp. ground black pepper
- ¼ tsp. kosher salt
- ¼ tsp. seasoned salt
- 2 tbsp. olive oil
- 5 tbsp. plain breadcrumbs
- 2 tbsp. panko breadcrumbs
- 2 tbsp. grated Parmesan cheese

Directions:

1. Preheat the Air Fryer to 380°F and grease. Season the chicken with pepper, kosher salt, and seasoned salt; set aside. In a bowl, pour olive oil. In a separate bowl, add crumb, and Parmesan cheese.

2. Place the chicken pieces in the oil to coat, then dip into breadcrumb mixture, and transfer to the Air Fryer. Work in batches if needed. Lightly spray chicken with cooking spray.
3. Cook the chicken for 10 minutes, flipping once halfway through. Cook until golden brown on the outside and no pinker on the inside.

Nutrition:

Calories 312, Fat 8.9g, Carbs 7g, Protein 10g

Butternut Squash with Thyme

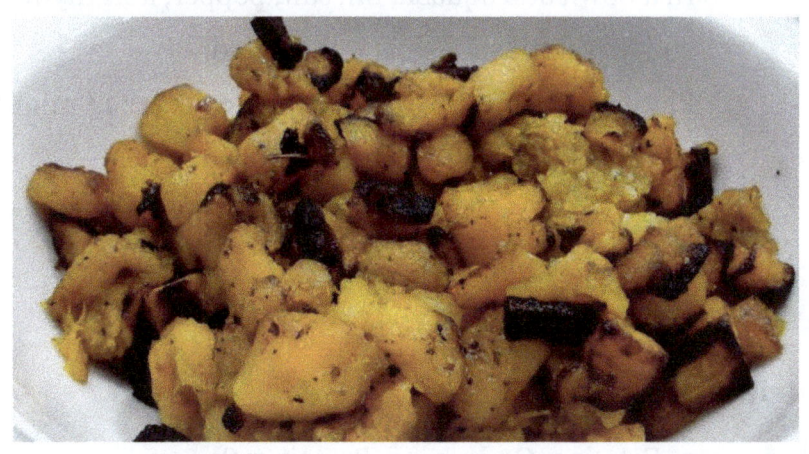

Preparation Time: 5 minutes

Cooking Time: 20 minutes:

Servings: 4

Ingredients:

- 2 cups peeled, butternut squash, cubed
- 1 tbsp. olive oil
- ¼ tsp. salt
- ¼ tsp. black pepper
- ¼ tsp. dried thyme
- 1 tbsp. finely chopped fresh parsley

Directions:

1. In a bowl, add squash, oil, salt, pepper, and thyme, and toss until squash is well-coated.
2. Place squash in the Air Fryer and cook for 14 minutes at 360°F.
3. When ready, sprinkle with freshly chopped parsley and serve chilled.

Nutrition:

Calories 219, Fat 4.3g, Carbs 9.4g, Protein 7.8

Chicken Breasts in Golden Crumb

Preparation Time: 10 minutes

Cooking Time: 25 minutes

Servings: 4

Ingredients:

- 1 ½ lb. chicken breasts, boneless, cut into strips
- 1 egg, lightly beaten
- 1 cup seasoned breadcrumbs
- Salt and black pepper to taste
- ½ tsp. dried oregano

Directions:

1. Preheat the Air Fryer to 390°F. Season the chicken with oregano, salt, and black pepper. In a small bowl, whisk in some salt and pepper to the beaten egg. In a separate bowl, add the crumbs. Dip chicken tenders in the egg wash, then in the crumbs.
2. Roll the strips in the breadcrumbs and press firmly, so the breadcrumbs stick well. Spray the chicken tenders with cooking spray and arrange them in the

Air Fryer. Cook for 14 minutes, until no longer pink in the center, and nice and crispy on the outside.

Nutrition:

Calories 223, Fat 3.2g, Carbs 4.3, Protein 5g

Yogurt Chicken Tacos

Preparation Time: 5 minutes

Cooking Time: 20 minutes:

Servings: 4

Ingredients:

- 1 cup cooked chicken, shredded
- 1 cup shredded mozzarella cheese
- ¼ cup salsa
- ¼ cup Greek yogurt
- Salt and ground black pepper
- 8 flour tortillas

Directions:

1. In a bowl, mix chicken, cheese, salsa, and yogurt, and season with salt and pepper. Spray one side of the tortilla with cooking spray. Lay 2 tbsp. of the chicken mixture at the center of the non-oiled side of each tortilla.
2. Roll tightly around the mixture. Arrange taquitos into your Air Fryer basket, without overcrowding. Cook in

batches if needed. Place the seam side down, or it will unravel during cooking crisps.

3. Cook it for 12 to 14 minutes, or until crispy, at 380°F.

Nutrition:

Calories 312, Fat 3g, Carbs 6.5g, Protein 6.2g

Flawless Kale Chips

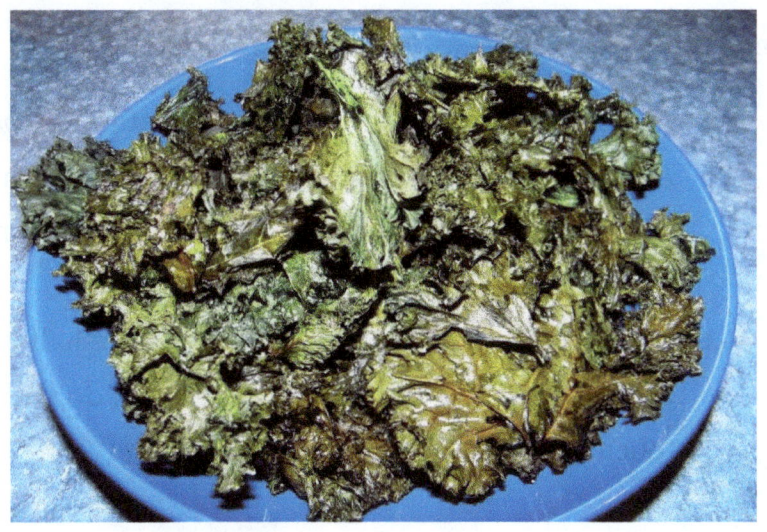

Preparation Time: 5 minutes

Cooking Time: 20 minutes:

Servings: 4

Ingredients:

- 4 cups chopped kale leaves; stems removed
- 2 tbsp. olive oil
- 1 tsp. garlic powder
- ½ tsp. salt
- ¼ tsp. onion powder

- ¼ tsp. black pepper

Directions:

1. In a bowl, mix kale and oil together, until well-coated. Add in garlic, salt, onion, and pepper and toss until well-coated. Arrange half the kale leaves to Air Fryer, in a single layer.
2. Cook for 8 minutes at 350°F, shaking once halfway through. Remove chips to a sheet to cool; do not touch.

Nutrition:

Calories 312, Fat 5.3g, Carbs 5g, Protein 7g

Vermicelli Noodles & Vegetables Rolls

Preparation Time: 5 minutes

Cooking Time: 25 minutes

Servings: 8

Ingredients:

- 8 spring roll wrappers
- 1 cup cooked and cooled vermicelli noodles
- 2 garlic cloves, finely chopped
- 1 tbsp. minced fresh ginger
- 2 tbsp. soy sauce
- 1 tsp. sesame oil
- 1 red bell pepper, seeds removed, chopped
- 1 cup finely chopped mushrooms
- 1 cup finely chopped carrot
- ½ cup finely chopped scallions

Directions:

1. In a saucepan, add garlic, ginger, soy sauce, pepper, mushroom, carrot and scallions, and stir-fry over

high heat for a few minutes, until soft. Add in vermicelli noodles; remove from the heat.
2. Place the spring roll wrappers onto a working board. Spoon the dollops of veggie and noodle mixture at the center of each spring roll wrapper. Roll the spring rolls and tuck the corners and edges in to create neat and secure rolls.
3. Spray with oil and transfer them to the Air Fryer. Cook for 12 minutes at 340°F, turning once halfway through. Cook until golden and crispy. Serve with soy or sweet chili sauce.

Nutrition:

Calories 312, Fat 5g, Carbs 5.4g, Protein 3g

Cheese Fish Balls

Preparation Time: 5 minutes

Cooking Time: 40 minutes

Servings: 6

Ingredients:

- 1 cup smoked fish, flaked
- 2 cups cooked rice
- 2 eggs, lightly beaten
- 1 cup grated Grana Padano cheese
- ¼ cup finely chopped thyme
- Salt and black pepper to taste
- 1 cup panko crumbs

Directions:

1. In a bowl, add fish, rice, eggs, Parmesan cheese, thyme, salt and pepper into a bowl; stir to combine. Shape the mixture into 12 even-sized balls. Roll the balls in the crumbs then spray with oil.
2. Arrange the balls into the fryer and cook for 16 minutes at 400°F, until crispy.

Nutrition:

Calories 234, Fat 5.2g, Carbs 4.3g, Protein 6.2g

Beef Balls with Mixed Herbs

Preparation Time: 5 minutes

Cooking Time: 25 minutes

Servings: 4

Ingredients:

- 1 lb. ground beef
- 1 onion, finely chopped
- 3 garlic cloves, finely chopped
- 2 eggs
- 1 cup breadcrumbs
- ½ cup fresh mixed herbs
- 1tbsp. mustard
- Salt and black pepper to taste
- Olive oil

Directions:

1. In a bowl, add beef, onion, garlic, eggs, crumbs, herbs, mustard, salt, and pepper and mix with hands to combine.

2. Shape into balls and arrange them in the Air Fryer's basket. Drizzle with oil and cook for 16 minutes at 380°F, turning once halfway through.

Nutrition:

Calories 315, Fat 5g, Carbs 9g, Protein 8g

Roasted Pumpkin Seeds

Preparation Time: 10 minutes

Cooking Time: 40 minutes

Servings: 4

Ingredients:

- 1 cup pumpkin seeds, pulp removed, rinsed
- 1 tbsp. butter, melted
- 1 tbsp. brown sugar
- 1 tsp. orange zest
- ½ tsp. cardamom
- ½ tsp. salt

Directions:

1. Cook the seeds for 4 minutes at 320°F, in your Air Fryer, to avoid moisture. In a bowl, whisk melted butter, sugar, zest, cardamom and salt.
2. Add the seeds to the bowl and toss to coat thoroughly.

3. Transfer the seeds to the Air Fryer and cook for 35 minutes at 300°F, shaking the basket every 10-12 minutes Cook until lightly browned.

Nutrition:

Calories 536, Fat 13g, Carbs 5g, Protein 7g

Buttery Parmesan Broccoli Florets

Preparation Time: 5 minutes

Cooking Time: 20 minutes:

Servings: 2

Ingredients:

- 2 tbsp. butter, melted
- 1 egg white
- 1 garlic clove, grated
- ¼ tsp. salt
- A pinch of black pepper
- ½ lb. broccoli florets
- ⅓ cup grated Parmesan cheese

Directions:

1. In a bowl, whisk together the butter, egg, garlic, salt, and black pepper.
2. Toss in broccoli to coat well.
3. Top with Parmesan cheese and; toss to coat.
4. Arrange broccoli in a single layer in the Air Fryer, without overcrowding.

5. Cook it in batches for 10 minutes at 360°F.
6. Remove to a serving plate and sprinkle with Parmesan cheese.

Nutrition:

Calories 350, Fat 27g, Carbs 20g, Protein 15 g

Spicy Chickpeas

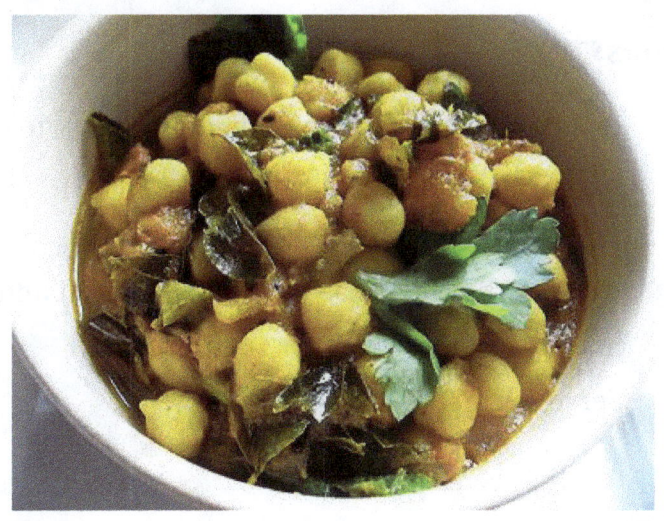

Preparation Time: 5 minutes

Cooking Time: 10 minutes

Servings: 4

Ingredients:

- 1 (15-oz.) can chickpeas rinsed and Dry-out
- 1 tbsp. olive oil
- ½ tsp. ground cumin
- ½ tsp. cayenne pepper
- ½ tsp. smoked paprika

- Salt, as required

Directions:

1. In a bowl, add all the ingredients and toss to coat well.
2. Preheat the Air Fryer at 390°F.
3. Arrange the chickpeas in Air Fryer basket and insert in the Air Fryer. Cook for 10 minutes.
4. Serve warm.

Nutrition:

Calories 146, Fat 4.5g, Carbs 18.8g, Protein 6.3g

Roasted Peanuts

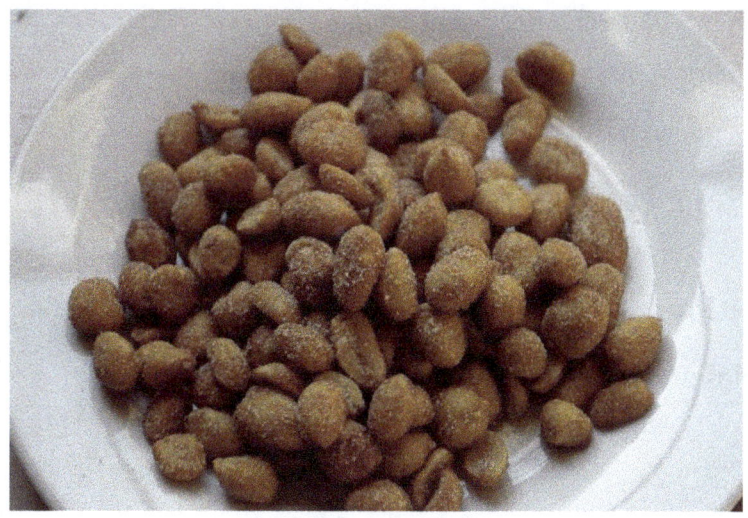

Preparation Time: 5 minutes

Cooking Time: 14 minutes

Servings: 6

Ingredients:

- 1½ cups raw peanuts
- Nonstick cooking spray

Directions:

1. Preheat the Air Fryer at 320°F.

2. Arrange the peanuts in Air Fryer basket and insert in the Air Fryer. Cook for 14 minutes.
3. Toss the peanuts twice.
4. After 9 minutes of cooking, spray the peanuts with cooking spray.
5. Serve warm.

Nutrition:

Calories 207, Fat 18g, Carbs 5.9g, Protein 9.4g

Roasted Cashews

Preparation Time: 5 minutes

Cooking Time: 5 minutes

Servings: 6

Ingredients:

- 1½ cups raw cashew nuts
- 1 tsp. butter, melted
- Salt and freshly ground black pepper, as needed

Directions:

1. In a bowl, mix together all the ingredients.
2. Preheat the Air Fryer at 355°F.
3. Arrange the cashew in Air Fryer basket and insert in the Air Fryer. Cook for 5 minutes.
4. Shake the cashews once halfway through.

Nutrition:

Calories 202, Fat 16.5g, Carbs 11.2g, Protein 5.3g

French Fries

Preparation Time: 15 minutes

Cooking Time: 30 minutes

Servings: 4

Ingredients:

- 1 lb. potatoes, peeled and cut into strips
- 3 tbsp. olive oil
- ½ tsp. onion powder
- ½ tsp. garlic powder
- 1 tsp. paprika

Directions:

1. In a large bowl of water, soak the potato strips for about 1 hour.
2. Dry out the potato strips well and pat them dry with the paper towels.
3. In a large bowl, add the potato strips and the remaining ingredients and toss to coat well.
4. Preheat the Air Fryer at 370°F.

5. Arrange the potatoe fries in Air Fryer basket and insert in the Air Fryer. Cook for 30 minutes.
6. Serve warm.

Nutrition:

Calories 172, Fat 10.7g, Carbs 18.6g, Protein 2.1g

Zucchini Fries

Preparation Time: 10 minutes

Cooking Time: 1 2 minutes

Servings: 4

Ingredients:

- 1 lb. zucchini, sliced into 2½-inch sticks
- Salt, as required
- 2 tbsp. olive oil
- ¾ cup panko breadcrumbs

Directions:

1. In a colander, add the zucchini and sprinkle with salt. Set aside for about 10 minutes. Gently pat dry the zucchini sticks with the paper towels and coat with oil.
2. In a shallow dish, add the breadcrumbs. Coat the zucchini sticks with breadcrumbs evenly.
3. Preheat the Air Fryer at 400°F.
4. Arrange the pan in Air Fryer basket and insert in the oven. Cook for 12 minutes.

5. Serve warm.

Nutrition:

Calories 151, Fat 8.6g, Carbs 6.9g, Protein 1.9g

Spicy Carrot Fries

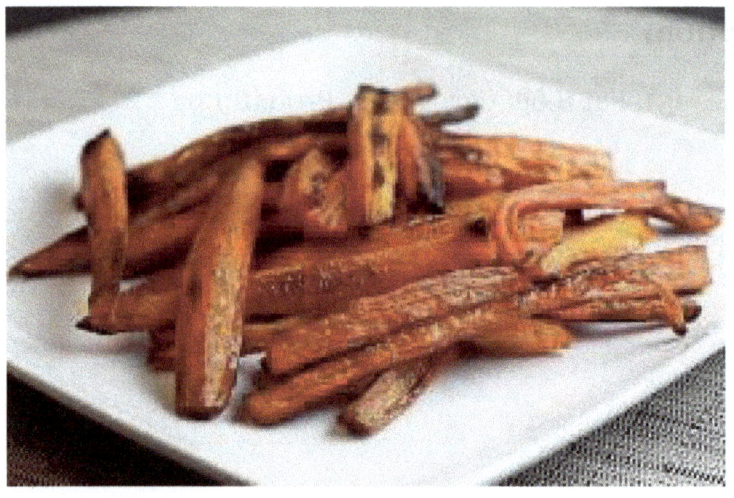

Preparation Time: 10 minutes

Cooking Time: 12 minutes

Servings: 2

Ingredients:

- 1 large carrot, peeled and cut into sticks
- 1 tbsp. fresh rosemary, chopped finely
- 1 tbsp. olive oil
- ¼ tsp. cayenne pepper
- Salt and ground black pepper, as required

Directions:

1. In a bowl, add all the ingredients and mix well.
2. Preheat the Air Fryer at 390°F.
3. Arrange the pan in Air Fryer basket and insert in the oven. Cook for 12 minutes.
4. Serve warm.

Nutrition:

Calories 81, Fat 8.3g, Carbs 4.7g, Protein 0.4g

Cinnamon Carrot Fries

Preparation Time: 10 minutes

Cooking Time: 12 minutes

Servings: 6

Ingredients:

- 1 lb. carrots, peeled and cut into sticks
- 1 tsp. maple syrup
- 1 tsp. olive oil
- ½ tsp. ground cinnamon
- Salt, to taste

Directions:

1. In a bowl, add all the ingredients and mix well.
2. Preheat the Air Fryer at 400°F.
3. Arrange the pan in Air Fryer basket and insert in the oven. Cook for 12 minutes.
4. Serve warm.

Nutrition:

Calories 41, Fat 0.8g, Carbs 8.3g, Protein 0.6g

Squash Fries

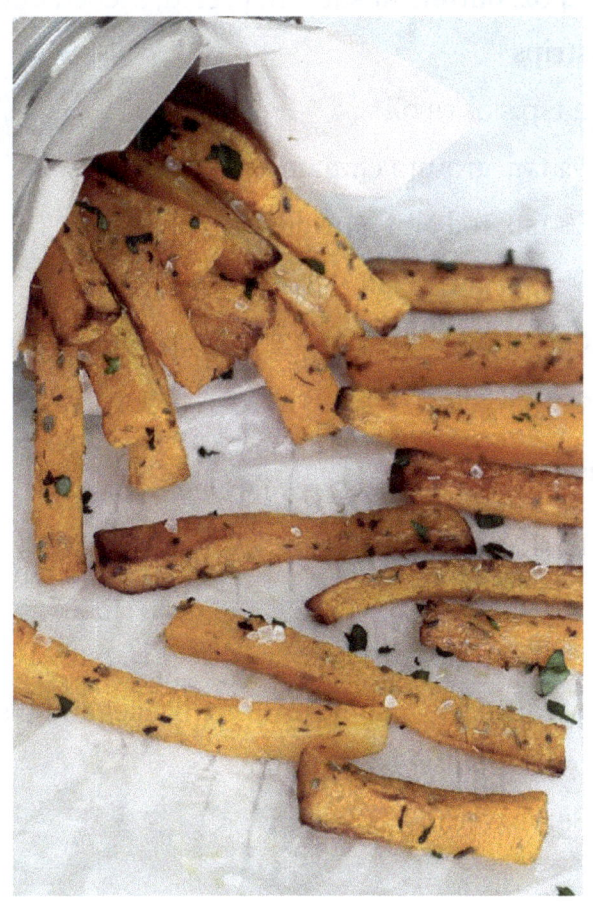

Preparation Time: 10 minutes

Cooking Time: 35 minutes

Servings: 2

Ingredients:

- 14 oz. butternut squash, peeled, seeded and cut into strips
- 2 tsp.s olive oil
- ½ tsp. ground cinnamon
- ½ tsp. red chili powder
- ¼ tsp. garlic salt
- Salt and freshly ground black pepper, as needed

Directions:

1. In a bowl, add all the ingredients and toss to coat well.
2. Preheat the Air Fryer at 400°F.
3. Arrange the pan in Air Fryer basket and insert in the oven. Cook for 30 minutes.
4. Serve warm.

Nutrition:

Calories 134, Fat 5g, Carbs 24.3g, Protein 2.1g

Avocado Fries

Preparation Time: 15 minutes

Cooking Time: 7 minutes

Servings: 2

Ingredients:

- ¼ cup all-purpose flour
- Salt and freshly ground black pepper, as needed
- 1 egg 1 tsp. water
- ½ cup panko breadcrumbs
- 1 avocado, peeled, pitted and sliced into 8 pieces
- Non-stick cooking spray

Directions:

1. In a shallow bowl, mix together the flour, salt, and black pepper.
2. In a second bowl, mix well egg and water.
3. In a third bowl, put the breadcrumbs.
4. Coat the avocado slices with flour mixture, then dip into egg mixture and finally, coat evenly with the breadcrumbs.

5. Now, spray the avocado slices evenly with cooking spray.
6. Preheat the Air Fryer at 400°F.
7. Arrange the pan in Air Fryer basket and insert in the oven. Cook for 7 minutes.
8. Serve warm.

Nutrition:

Calories 340, Fat 14g, Carbs 30g, Protein 23g

Dill Pickle Fries

Preparation Time: 15 minutes

Cooking Time: 15 minutes

Servings: 8

Ingredients:

- 1 (16-oz.) jar spicy dill pickle spears Dry out and pat dried
- ¾ cup all-purpose flour
- ½ tsp. paprika
- 1 egg, beaten
- ¼ cup milk
- 1 cup panko breadcrumbs
- Nonstick cooking spray

Directions:

1. In a shallow dish, mix together the flour, and paprika.
2. In a second dish, place the milk and egg and mix well.
3. In a third dish, put the breadcrumbs.

4. Coat the pickle spears with flour mixture, then dip into egg mixture and finally, coat evenly with the breadcrumbs.
5. Now, spray the pickle spears evenly with cooking spray.
6. Preheat the Air Fryer at 400°F.
7. Arrange the pan in Air Fryer basket and insert in the oven. Cook for 15 minutes.
8. Serve warm.
9. Flip the fries once halfway through.
10. Serve warm.

Nutrition:

Calories 110, Fat 1.9g, Carbs 12.8g, Protein 2.7g

Mozzarella Sticks

Preparation Time: 15 minutes

Cooking Time: 12 minutes

Servings: 3

Ingredients:

- ¼ cup white flour
- 2 eggs
- 3 tbsp. nonfat milk
- 1 cup plain breadcrumbs
- 1 lb. Mozzarella cheese block cut into 3x½-inch sticks

Directions:

1. In a shallow dish, add the flour.
2. In a second shallow dish, mix together the eggs, and milk.
3. In a third shallow dish, place the breadcrumbs.
4. Coat the Mozzarella sticks with flour, then dip into egg mixture and finally, coat evenly with the breadcrumbs.

5. Preheat the Air Fryer at 400°F.
6. Arrange the pan in Air Fryer basket and insert in the oven. Cook for 12 minutes.
7. Serve warm

Nutrition:

Calories 254, Fat 6.6g, Carbs 35.2g, Protein 12.8g

Tortilla Chips

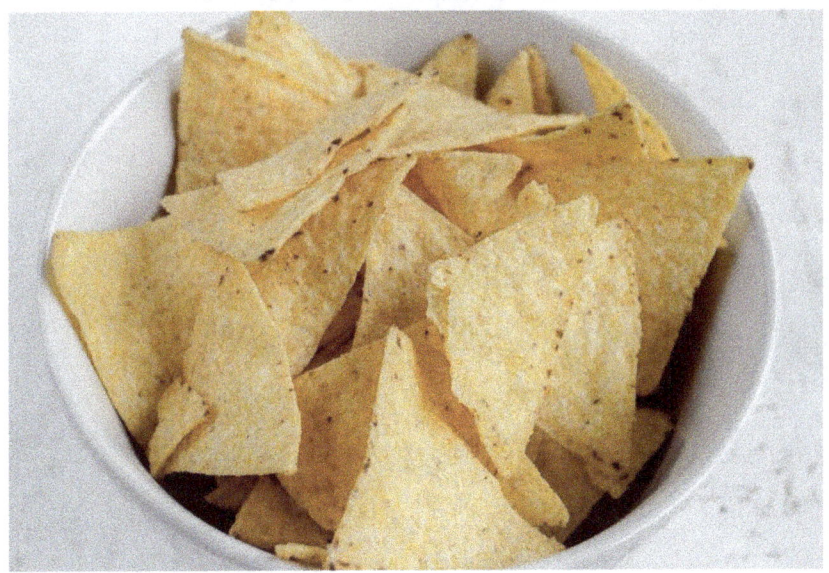

Preparation Time: 10 minutes

Cooking Time: 3 minutes

Servings: 3

Ingredients:

- 4 corn tortillas cut into triangles
- 1 tbsp. olive oil
- Salt, to taste

Directions:

1. Coat the tortilla chips with oi and then, sprinkle each side of the tortillas with salt.
2. Preheat the Air Fryer at 390°F.
3. Arrange the pan in Air Fryer basket and insert in the oven. Cook for 3 minutes.
4. Serve warm.

Nutrition:

Calories 110, Fat 5.6g, Carbs 14.3g, Protein 1.8g

Sky-High Roasted Corn

Preparation Time: 5 minutes

Cooking Time: 10 minutes

Servings: 4

Ingredients:

- 4 ears of husk-less corn
- 1 tbsp. of olive oil
- 1 tsp. of salt
- 1 tsp. of black pepper

Directions:

1. Heat up your Air Fryer to 400°F.
2. Sprinkle the ears of corn with the olive oil, salt and black pepper.
3. Place it inside your Air Fryer and cook it for 10 minutes at 400°F.
4. Serve and enjoy!

Nutrition:

Calories 100, Fat 1g, Carbs 22g, Protein 3g

Ravishing Air-Fried Carrots with Honey Glaze

Preparation Time: 5 minutes

Cooking Time: 10 minutes

Servings: 1

Ingredients:

- 3 cups of chopped into ½-inch pieces carrots
- 1 tbsp. of olive oil
- 2 tbsp. of honey
- 1 tbsp. of brown sugar
- salt and black pepper

Directions:

1. Heat up your Air Fryer to 390°F.
2. Using a bowl, add and toss the carrot pieces, olive oil, honey, brown sugar, salt, and the black pepper until it is properly covered.
3. Place it inside your Air Fryer and add the seasoned glazed carrots.

4. Cook it for 12 minutes at a 390°F, and then shake after 6 minutes. Serve and enjoy!

Nutrition:

Calories 90, Fat 3.5g, Carbs 13g, Protein 1g

Flaming Buffalo Cauliflower Bites

Preparation Time: 5 minutes

Cooking Time: 20 minutes:

Servings: 4

Ingredients:

- 1 large chopped into florets cauliflower head
- 3 beaten eggs
- 2/3 cup of cornstarch
- 2 tbsp. of melted butter
- ¼ cup of hot sauce

Directions:

1. Heat up your Air Fryer to 360°F.
2. Using a large mixing bowl, add and mix the eggs and the cornstarch properly.
3. Add the cauliflower, gently toss it until it is properly covered with the batter, shake it off in case of any excess batter and set it aside.

4. Grease your Air Fryer basket with a nonstick cooking spray and add the cauliflower bites which will require you to work in batches.
5. Cook the cauliflower bites for 15 to 20 minutes: or until it has a golden-brown color and a crispy texture, while still shaking occasionally.
6. Then, using a small mixing bowl, add and mix the melted butter and hot sauce properly.
7. Once the cauliflower bites are done, remove it from your Air Fryer and place it into a large bowl. Pour the buffalo sauce over the cauliflower bites and toss it until it is properly covered.
8. Serve and enjoy!

Nutrition:

Calories 240, Fat 5.5g, Carbs 37g, Protein 8.8g

Pleasant Air-Fried Eggplant

Preparation Time: 5 minutes

Cooking Time: 20 minutes:

Servings: 4

Ingredients:

- 2 thinly sliced or chopped into chunks eggplants
- 1 tsp. of salt
- 1 tsp. of black pepper
- 1 cup of rice flour
- 1 cup of white wine

Directions:

1. Using a bowl, add the rice flour, white wine and mix properly until it gets smooth.
2. Add the salt, black pepper and stir again.
3. Dredge the eggplant slices or chunks into the batter and remove any excess batter.
4. Heat up your Air Fryer to 390°F.
5. Grease your Air Fryer basket with a nonstick cooking spray.

6. Add the eggplant slices or chunks into your Air Fryer and cook it for 15 to 20 minutes: or until it has a golden brown and crispy texture, while still shaking it occasionally.
7. Carefully remove it from your Air Fryer and allow it to cool off. Serve and enjoy!

Nutrition:

Calories 380, Fat 15g, Carbs 51g, Protein 13g

www.ingramcontent.com/pod-product-compliance
Lightning Source LLC
Chambersburg PA
CBHW071107030426
42336CB00013BA/1985